Manage High Blood Pressure Naturally

Manage your blood pressure naturally and stop taking medicines

By

V.K.Grover

Why you need this book

According to the American Heart Association (AHA), about 65 million Americans over the age of 20 have high blood pressure. That is about one in three adults in the United States. Only about 63 percent of those with high blood pressure are only aware that they have it.

The reasons so many people do not know they have high blood pressure, also known as hypertension, is that there are not really any clear symptoms of hypertension. In fact, according to the AHA, the cause of 90 to 95 percent of the cases of high blood pressure in America is not known.

So why should a person worry if he or she has high blood pressure? Hypertension raises your risk for other health problems, including heart attacks and strokes. In 2010, more than 52,000 Americans died because of complications related to high blood pressure. The rate of death from high blood pressure increased nearly 30 percent between 1993 and 2004.

It is important that we should get our blood pressure tested regularly and take corrective action if it is high. In fact we should take proper food and do exercise so that the B.P is under control. Often the only way a person finds out that they have high blood pressure is when their blood pressure is tested.
Doctors have a variety of drugs in their arsenals to try but all of them have side effects.
Doctors use following types of medicines for treatment of high blood pressure.

Diuretics, Beta Blockers, and Ace Inhibitors.

All these medicines have side effects. The main problem with diuretics is that they cannot distinguish between flushing out things that are good for the body and things that are bad. In addition to getting rid of excess water and salt, they can also rid your body of nutrients that might be helpful in lowering your blood pressure. Potassium is an example, which is an important ingredient for lowering of blood pressure.

Diuretics remove many other electrolytes like calcium, potassium etc besides sodium, and that can cause weakness, dizziness and irregular heartbeat, among other problems.

Side effects of beta blockers can include insomnia, cold hands and feet, tiredness and depression. People who have diabetes need to be monitored very carefully if they are taking insulin along with beta blockers. They increase asthma symptoms, lowered good cholesterol levels or an increased heart rate while side effects of ACE inhibitors include skin rashes, loss of your sense of taste, or a chronic, dry cough. In rare instances kidney damage can also occur.

Because of these side effects it is better to control High Blood pressure through natural means which include changes in life style, diet, proper exercise, and use of herbs. This book helps you in managing your blood pressure through natural means without any side effects and remains healthy.

DISCLAIMER AND/OR LEGAL NOTICES

My efforts through this book are to let the readers know the limitless values of alternative/natural medicines. I have observed that these simple and cheap methods of cure can go a long way for treatment of Blood Pressure.

The information within this book is intended as reference materials only and not as medical or professional advice. Information contained herein is intended to give you the tools to make informed decisions about your lifestyle and health. It should not be used as a substitute for any treatment that has been prescribed or recommended by your doctor. The information presented herein represents the views of the author.

Thanks

I am grateful to God who inspired me to write this book.

I am also thankful to my wife and children and friends for their love and support, without which it would not have been possible to write this book.

Contents

Chapter no.	contents	Page
1	Introduction	8
2	How B.P is maintained	11
3	Types and causes of High Blood pressure	13
4	Risk factors for High Blood Pressure	17
5	Effect of medicines used for bringing down Blood pressure.	20
6	Natural methods for treatment of High Blood Pressure	25
7	Food	30
8	Electrolytes and B.P	36
9	Effect of Molecular Wastes/Free Radicals on blood pressure	44
10	Ayurveda and Blood Pressure	47
11	The High Blood Pressure Natural Remedies	50
12.	Other natural methods	57
13	Annexure1 Characteristics of A Type behaviour	65
14.	Annexure2 Meditation Method	67
15.	Annexure 3 Copper/Silver/Gold and Iron charged water	70

Chapter 1

Introduction

What is Blood Pressure

Blood pressure is basically the force exerted on the arteries by the blood as it passes through them. Someone with high blood pressure has blood that is putting higher-than- normal pressure on the arteries, which puts more stress on the body.

The heart has to work so hard to get the blood pumped through those arteries that it can actually enlarge and damage the heart, eventually causing heart attacks, strokes, aneurysm and other heart problems if left untreated.

A healthy heart usually beats 6o to 70 times per minute when a person is at rest. The blood pressure is different depending on whether the heart is beating or is at rest. A blood pressure reading is actually a measurement of both of these numbers.

The measure of blood pressure while the heart is beating is known as systolic pressure, while the pressure when the heart is at rest is called diastolic pressure. Your blood pressure when measured, is reported as one number "over" another, such as 12o/80. The top number is your systolic pressure, while the bottom is your diastolic pressure.

The actual measuring of blood pressure is done with the help of a blood pressure tester. Earlier the B.P was measured by doctors using blood pressure cuff. Now B.P can be measured by anyone using Digital B.P. Tester.
Blood pressure cuff includes a cuff that is secured around the upper arm, and two rubber tubes--one of which goes to the rubber bulb that inflates the cuff, and the other which goes to a reservoir containing mercury. The effect of the pressure on the mercury is actually how the blood pressure is measured.

As air is blown into the cuff, the doctor or nurse taking your blood pressure will listen for the pulse. When he or she first hears the pulse, the systolic measurement is recorded. When the sound of the pulse recedes, the doctor or nurse then takes the diastolic reading. The unit of measure is actually millimeters of mercury, reflecting the use of mercury in the test.

Principle of measuring B.P by Digital tester is similar but here the air pressure is given by the built in pump and B.P measured automatically by using digital instrument.

While measuring B.P BY Digital instrument care should be taken that the cuff is 4 to 5 mm from the elbow and is at height of the heart. This is required to get correct reading.

When we visit the doctor for measurement of B.P, we are normally under tension and this leads to higher B.P. This phenomenon is known as "White Coat Blood Pressure."

A blood pressure reading reflects what our B.P is at the moment. Throughout the day it keeps fluctuating.

It increases during period of activity, when our heart has to work harder, such as when we exercise and decreases when we are at rest when there is less demand on our heart as when we sleep.

The daily or even hourly ups and downs are perfectly normal. It is normally the highest in the morning hours after we are awake and become active. This is one of the reasons that doctors usually recommend to take BP medicine in the morning so that peak in BP can be avoided.

Best period for taking BP is during the day after you have been active for a few hours.

If you are doing exercise, it is better to measure before hand or several hours afterwards. After physical activity, BP remains at low level for 1-2 hours.

You should not smoke; drink coffee or alcohol at least 30 minutes before taking B.P.

Go to wash room before taking BP as full bladder increases the BP.

WHAT IS CONSIDERED HIGH BLOOD PRESSURE?

You may not be knowing what normal or High B.P reading are.

Here are the numbers what is usually considered "normal," as well as prehypertension and hypertension.

	Systolic	Diastolic
Normal	Less than 120	Less than 80
Prehypertension	120-139	80-89
Stage One	140-159	90-99
Stage Two	160 or higher	100 or higher

These numbers are considered the proper range for adults who are not on blood pressure medication and do not have illnesses such as kidney disease. If your blood pressure does not clearly fall into one of these categories, the higher number is the decisive number to look at. For instance, if your systolic blood pressure is 125, but your diastolic is 75, you would still be considered prehypertension.

Of course one high reading does not mean that you have high blood pressure. Your blood pressure could be high because you are stressed out or because of a medication you are taking, so you would have to see a trend of high blood pressure readings to consider yourself as having high blood pressure.

Chapter 2

How is BP maintained?

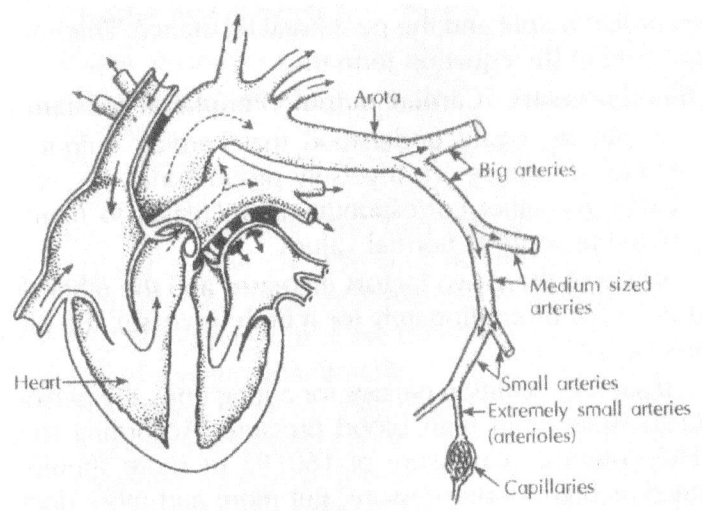

Fig1: Heart and arteries

Heart is special natural pump made up of special muscles. It incessantly and rhythmically beats maintaining the blood-circulation. Usually, it beats 72 times a minute. This number is termed, the 'heart rate'. At every contraction, the heart pumps about 70 ml (half a cup) of blood into the arteries. This quantity is termed, the °stroke volume'.

Thus it pumps about 5 litres of blood every minute. This quantity is termed, the 'cardiac output'. This can be expressed in the equation form thus:

Cardiac output = Stroke volume x Heart rate

The main artery, the aorta, arising from the heart divides into branches. These branches, in turn, give rise to smaller and smaller arteries. Such branching finally gives rise to extremely small arteries called 'arterioles'. The walls of the arterioles possess muscle fibers. The arterioles can, therefore, contract or expand as per the bodily needs. Usually the arterioles possess a tone i.e., they remain in a partially contracted state, thus slowing down the flow of blood. Such resistance to the flow of blood by the arterioles is called 'peripheral resistance'.

Blood pressure is the result of the interaction between the cardiac output and the peripheral resistance. This can be expressed in the equation form as:

Blood pressure= Cardiac output x Peripheral resistance

It can be easily understood that cardiac output and peripheral resistance are inversely proportional, i.e., if one increases, the other correspondingly decreases to maintain the blood pressure at normal values.

If one of these two factors increases and the other does not decrease proportionately (or if both increase), the blood pressure goes up.

If such a condition persists for a long time, the person is said to suffer from high blood pressure. According to the WHO criterion, a pressure of 160/95 or more should be termed as high blood pressure. But more and more doctors now consider 140/90 also as high blood pressure. In the words of Dr. William Kannel, professor of internal medicine and chief of the hypertension unit at the University of Texas, Health Science Center at Dallas Kannel, "lower the pressure, the better for a person"

Chapter 3

Types and causes of High Blood pressure

There are two types of High Blood Pressures
a) Essential (simple) and
b) Secondary
Secondary high blood pressure is caused by some other disease in the body like problem of liver, kidney.
More than 90% of patients suffer from essential hypertension. What changes or mechanisms in the body cause hypertension is not clear but some reasons are given here.

Reasons for high blood pressure

- Heredity: If your parents had high blood pressure, you are more likely to have it as well. Some experts believe that incidence of High BP is double in kins of persons with high BP than normal persons but other researchers believe that it is not hereditary but environmental factors that cause High B.P. As the children eat the same food as their parents, they also get high BP. What way and to what extent do hereditary factors act, is not clear. In short, it can be said if exciting environmental forces are not at play, heredity can have little influence.
- Mental tension and negative thinking: All researchers accept the role of mental tension and negative thinking in the development of high blood pressure.

Mental tension leads to excessive secretion of catecholamine (adrenaline and nor-adrenaline) inside the body. These secretions undesirably stimulate atecholaminergic nerve endings in the brain-stem to cause an elevation of the blood pressure.

The incidence of high blood pressure in too ambitious, too much self-controlled or emotion-throttling (who consciously refrain from expressing their feelings) and workaholic persons, has been found to be much higher.

Studies and widespread surveys have shown that persons with a particular type of personality or behaviour-pattern suffer from high blood pressure more often. Scientists have named such behaviour: 'type A behaviour'. Type A behaviour has clear cut characteristics.

To avoid high B.P, the reader should try to avoid to be A type person as 'type A' person normally attracts high blood pressure and coronary heart disease.

Mental tension or 'type A' personality stimulates the secretion of certain undesirable juices inside the body, which increase the arteriolar resistance and cause high blood pressure.

(Characteristics of A Type persons are given in Annexure 1.)

Other reasons that can cause high B.P are

• Race: African Americans are more likely than Caucasians to have high blood pressure.
• Gender: Men are more likely than women to have high blood pressure.
• Age: As you get older, your risk increases

• Refined Salt Intake: It is mentioned that sodium affects blood pressure, but it is observed that it is not quantity of sodium but higher ratio of sodium to potassium, calcium and magnesium that increases high B.P. Most people get much more sodium than they need. It is felt that people should take only one tea spoon of salt daily to keep B.P. in control. Instead of using refined salts try sea salts or rock salts that contain other minerals like potassium, calcium also. Avoid any pre-packaged, high-salt foods.

• Obesity: Being overweight is a huge risk factor for high blood pressure. After examining 74000 industrial workers, Dr. Master, Dublin, and Marks found that B.P is proportional to body weight.

The greater the obesity, the higher the B.P. It is also observed that in obese, higher pressure develops much earlier in life.

• Smoking: Robs your heart of oxygen and can increase B.P.
• Living a sedentary lifestyle: The incidence of high blood pressure is much higher in sedentary persons than in physical labourers.

In a study covering 1000 athletes, it was found that they had a systolic pressure of only 99 mm Hg on an average.

In addition, there are other factors or conditions that can increase your risk of high blood pressure, including:

- Being pregnant;
- Having diabetes;
- Drinking alcohol to excess: (How so ever small quantities of alcohol are good for B.P.) and
- Taking oral contraceptives or other medications such as steroids, diet pills, cold remedies.

causes of secondary High Blood pressure.

Secondary High BP is more serious and can be due to some physical problem.

	Cause/Type	Symptoms	Investigations	Treatment
1	Co-arctation (kinking) of the aorta	Headache, weakness of leg muscles, varicose veins on the back and waist, etc. The blood pressure in arm-arteries is high but that in leg-arteries is normal or low.	X ray, E C G	Surgery
2	A disorder of kidney/s (e.g., glomerulonephritis, pyelone-phritis, systemic lupus anythymatosus, poly-arteritis nodosa, polycystic kidney, renal artery stenosis, etc.)	Onset in very young or very old age; pain in the abdomen and the back; peculiar sounds (bruits) in the abdomen on asculfation; an absence of family history.	Urine, I. V. P., etc.	In some disorders surgery may help
3	Hormonal imbalance or long term use of hormone drugs (disorders include pheochromocytoma, Cushing's syndrome, aldosteronism and use of contraceptive pills)	History of consumption of contraceptive pills; excessive muscle-weakness; hair on the face in women; moon-like face, etc. Patients with pheochromocytoma get attacks of sweating and headache.	X Ray photographs of bones; chemical tests to determine the concentrations of hormones in the blood; urine analysis to determine concen-trations of V. M. A.; X-Ray abdomen	Stop using contraceptive pills or hormone drugs; In some disorders; surgery or medicines may help
4	Pregnancy (pressure becomes high in only some pregnant women, not all)	None except elevation of pressure	None	Medicines
5	Long term use of drugs called mono-amino oxidase inhibitors.	None except elevation of pressure	None	Stop using the culprit drugs.

Chapter 4

RISK FACTORS FOR HIGH BLOOD PRESSURE

Since symptoms of High BP are not always clear it is better to look at risk factors that high blood pressure can cause.

- High blood pressure adds to the workload of the heart and arteries. It may contribute to heart failure, strokes, kidney disorders, and arteriosclerosis. The narrowed blood vessels are squeezed and cannot deliver enough oxygen and nutrients to the body's organs, muscles, and tissues.
- Enlarged heart. When the heart is forced to work harder than normal for a long period of time, it becomes enlarged. Although a slightly enlarged heart may function well, a heart that is very much enlarged has a difficult time keeping up with demands of daily living.

- Wear and tear. Arteries and arterioles show the wear and tear of high blood pressure. Eventually, they become hardened, less elastic, and scarred. High blood pressure accelerates this dangerous reaction.

- Life-threatening risks. Hardened or narrowed arteries cannot deliver required amounts of blood, oxygen, and nutrients to body's organs.

A blood clot may also lodge in a narrowed artery, depriving part of the body its normal blood supply. The three vital organs most frequently damaged are the heart, brain, and kidneys.

Details of risks in detail are given below

(1) Atherosclerosis (hardening of the blood vessels)
The blood vessels of a healthy person are highly elastic. This property of elasticity is extremely essential because organs require less or more blood as per the need of the situation For example, heart requires more blood when a person is doing a strenuous activity. At such a time, the coronary arteries expand so as to carry more blood to the heart.

High blood pressure renders the blood vessel narrow and hard.Narrow and hardened arteries cannot expand to carry more blood even when necessary. Chest pain (angina pectoris) arises when coronary arteries supplying nutrition to the heart do not expand during physical activity.

In the case of atherosclerosis progressing unabated coronary artery may become too narrow and may get totally obstructed resulting into the death of a part the heart muscle which is heart attack.

(2) Heart failure: When blood pressure is high, the heart has to overwork. To perform the increased work, the heart muscle thickens and increases in size. For a period of time, despite the increased workload, the heart does well. It accommodates and handles the burden. But after certain time, it tires and is unable to fully meet the strain. The result is congestive heart failure.

In heart failure, the heart does not stop beating. It continues to beat but its contractions are no longer as complete and effective. With each contraction, less volume of blood is pumped.

There are many effects of loss of pumping efficiency or heart failure. Since less blood reaches the tissues of the body, muscles suffer from lack of adequate nourishment and there is muscle fatigue. Less blood may reach the brain and the patient may not be able to think as effectively as he previously could.

There is a build-up of pressure within the heart itself
Unable to pump out blood completely, the heart experiences increased internal pressure as its chambers dilate and become reservoirs for abnormal amounts of blood. The pressure extends backwards to the lungs, which may then retain fluids sometimes as much as several litres. From the lungs the pressure is transmitted still further back to the veins of the body, the liver and the legs. The liver becomes congested and enlarged; the legs swell with fluids; the neck vein becomes distended.

In spite of vigorous treatment, 50 per cent of persons suffering from heart failure do not survive for more than five years; and 20 per cent of them even die within a year.
An electrocardiogram (ECG) is helpful to make sure no damage has occurred to the heart. You may have even had a heart attack without realizing it. This test will show you how your heart is doing.

(3) Detrimental effects on kidneys: If the blood pressure is elevated, the kidneys cannot perform their work of blood-filtration effectively. Consequently salt and toxins accumulate in the body. Each gram of salt accumulated in the body has a capacity to hold back 70 grams of water from being excreted. Such water retention aggravates heart failure.

High blood pressure also gradually destroys the cells of the kidneys. Kidney damage is manifested by loss of useful nutrients through the urine. A study conducted by Dr. Perera showed that 42 per cent of people who did nothing to control their blood pressure, lost albumin in their urine. Statistics show that unless vigorously and incessantly treated, persons losing albumin in their urine do not survive for more than five years.

Blood may be taken to check for kidney disease, which can cause high blood pressure, as well as for abnormal vitamin and mineral levels, which could indicate a gland problem.

(4) Arteriolar inflammation: Some patients of high blood pressure suffer from inflammation of the arterioles. The cells of the walls of the arterioles undergo necrosis and destruction. The symptoms of this disorder include rapidly increasing high blood pressure (accelerated hypertension), retinal haemorrhages and progressive kidney failure. There was a time when arteriolar inflammation led to an almost certain death within a year. Today, however, a patient's life can be prolonged with effective drugs.

(5) Dissecting aneurysm of the aorta: A part of the main artery (aorta) becomes thin in some patients of high blood pressure. The cells of the thinned part undergo rotting and destruction. The thinned part may then balloon out either outwards or inwards (into the lumen of the aorta). If it balloons inwards, it obstructs the flow of blood. If it balloons outwards, it may rupture, causing massive haemorrhage. If the condition is immediately diagnosed, the patient's life may be saved by drugs and an operation; if not, death soon ensues.

(6) Reduced life-expectancy: The most serious hazard of high blood pressure is that it shortens life.

For example, for a man of 35, if the blood pressure is 142/85, the mortality rate is 150 per cent above average; if the blood pressure is 152/85, the mortality rate increases to 225 per cent; if the blood pressure is 145/95, the mortality rate is again 225 per cent above average; if the blood pressure is 152/95, the mortality rate increases to 300 per cent above average. This sixth risk factor indicates that however mild the elevation of blood pressure, zealous efforts should be made to bring it down, without delay.

Chapter 5

Effect of medicines used for bringing down Blood pressure.

Doctors have a variety of drugs in their arsenals to try but all of them have side effects. We discuss these medicines and their effects below.

DIURETICS

One of the most popular treatments for high blood pressure is a prescription diuretic.
These drugs remove fluid and salt from the body, which decreases the volume of blood in the body, allowing it to flow more easily through the blood vessels.
Because sensitivity to salt is sometimes to blame in high blood pressure cases, flushing out the salt and beginning a lower-salt diet can be helpful for those people who are actually sensitive to sodium.
The main problem with diuretics, however, is that they cannot distinguish between flushing out things that are good for the body and things that are bad.in addition to getting rid of excess water and salt, they can also rid your body of nutrients that might be helpful in lowering your blood pressure.
Potassium is a huge example, which is an important ingredient for lowering of blood pressure.
Diuretics remove many other electrolytes like calcium, potassium etc besides sodium, and that can cause weakness, dizziness and irregular heartbeat, among other problems.

BETA BLOCKERS

Another major category of blood pressure medication is known as beta blockers.

These drugs reduce the nerve impulses to the heart and blood vessels, making the heart beat more slowly and with less force. This causes the blood pressure to drop because the blood is putting less force on the vessels.

Side effects of beta blockers can include insomnia, cold hands and feet, tiredness and depression. People who have diabetes need to be monitored very carefully if they are taking insulin along with beta blockers.

If you have been taking beta blockers and then stop using them, you may have increased asthma symptoms, lowered good cholesterol levels or an increased heart rate. Beta blockers are a good example of why, if you use traditional medicine for your treatment of high blood pressure, you may end up having to take drugs for the rest of your life. The rebound when you go off the drugs can be dramatic.

ACE INHIBITORS

Angiotensin Converting Enzyme inhibitors, also known as ACE inhibitors, prevent the formation of a chemical, angiotensin II, which causes the blood vessels to narrow.

Taking an ACE inhibitor can help the blood vessels relax, allowing blood to flow easily.

Side effects of ACE inhibitors include skin rashes, loss of your sense of taste, or a chronic, dry cough. In rare instances kidney damage can also occur.

Other similar drugs include the angiotensin II receptor blockers—which shield blood vessels from angiotensin, allowing the blood vessels to widen—and calcium channel blockers, which keep calcium from moving into the muscle cells of the blood vessels and heart, allowing vessels to relax and blood pressure to go down.

Both of these types of drugs may cause dizziness, while the calcium channel blockers can also lead to heart palpitations, headaches, swollen ankles, constipation and varied other problems depending on the particular type of ACE inhibitor you are taking.

ALPHA BLOCKERS

Alpha blockers reduce nerve impulses to the blood vessels. Without the impulses, the muscles cannot contract. This relaxes the blood vessels, allowing blood to flow more easily and the blood pressure to be reduced.

When you first take an alpha blocker, you may have a huge dip in blood pressure that causes dizziness and can make you feel faint. After continued use of the drug, side effects may include headaches, nausea, and weakness, pounding heart, weight gain and increase of "bad" cholesterol. Some studies have even shown that alpha blockers can cause heart failure when used for long-term--exactly one of the conditions you are trying to prevent by treating your high blood pressure!

Sometimes alpha and beta blockers are combined to make for a safer treatment plan, but all of the same side effects and potential problems are still there.

VASODILATORS

Vasodilators, also known as blood vessel dilators, open the blood vessels by relaxing the muscle in the vessel walls, allowing blood pressure to go down. These drugs are usually used with other blood pressure reducing drugs for best results.
These drugs can cause headaches, swelling around the eyes, heart palpitations or aches and pains in the joints. These symptoms usually go away after a couple of weeks. One vasodilator you may have heard of is Minoxidil, which is also marketed as a hair-growth stimulator. It should not be a surprise, then, that a side effect of taking it for high blood pressure is hair growth. Another is extreme weight gain. It is only used in very severe cases of high blood pressure that do not respond to other treatments.

Some long term clinical studies have confirmed that taking of blood pressure prescription drugs cause unnecessary side effects such as fatigue, headaches, impotence, sleep disturbances and many more including increased risk of heart disease. Almost every known medical authority including the Joint National Committee on detection, evaluation, and treatment of High Blood Pressure has been recommending the use of non-drug therapies for treatment of mild High Blood Pressure. All of them agree that
- Drugs carry no benefit.
- They possess significant risk.

American Journal of Cardiology states that there is little evidence that patients with marginal hypertension will achieve enough benefit to justify the costs and adverse effects of antihypertensive drug treatment.

Dr. Julian Whitaker director of Whitaker Wellness Institute Newport Beach, California says, "Volumes of scientific research show that dietary changes can eliminate high blood pressure or hypertension in most patients. But most doctors start a patient on drugs without recommendations for dietary changes. The dangerous side effects of blood pressure drugs often make this approach, in my opinion, more harmful to the patients than beneficial".

These are only a few of the doctors/medical institutes that are not in favour of using blood pressure prescribed medicines for treating High Blood Pressure.

Norman Kaplan, M.D., professor of internal medicine and chief of the hypertension unit at the University of Texas Health Science Center at Dallas says:

"I believe a non-drug approach should be the first treatment of mild hypertension, where the diastolic blood pressure reading [lower number] is between 90 and 100 mm Hg, The steadily growing tendency to treat even mildly hypertensive patients with drugs is bringing millions of asymptomatic [without symptoms] people into lifetime drug therapy. For some, the risks of the drugs, as we have used them, may outweigh the benefits that can be gained from lowering the blood pressure. It is true that antihypertensive drugs will control blood pressure and that they have been shown to lower the death rate from stroke and heart failure that sometimes result from high blood pressure. But antihypertensive drugs have only spotty effects against what is by far the most serious and common complication of hypertension—coronary artery disease. I think we should consider all risk factors, along with the level of the blood pressure, before making the decision to use drugs."

Howsoever In today's health culture, synthetic treatments (pharmaceuticals) are readily prescribed to individuals to treat their symptoms and ease their discomfort. These synthetic treatments bring quick relief for the symptoms but typically leave the ailment untreated and treat only the symptoms, though Dr. Koppler believes that these medicines are not very harmful. But it is proved beyond doubt by research these substances often have side effects which further compromise the individual's health and may require treatment with additional substances.

Although allopathic medicine certainly has a role to play and has made a tremendous contribution to medical science during the past century, there is a growing perception that it is not the only answer and that, in many cases, holistic medicine can accomplish just as much, if not more--without the risk of side effects, addiction and sacrifice to health so commonly associated with pharmaceutical drugs.

Contrary to common perception natural medicines can work quickly and safely to promote healing. In many cases, they can succeed where pharmaceutical drugs have failed. Despite frequent reports that they are 'unproven' and 'untested', the opposite is true. Natural medicines have a long history of usage and there is a wealth of empirical evidence to support their effectiveness and safety. In addition, many academic hospitals and universities carry out active clinical research to support the extensive traditional and empirical evidence behind natural medicines.

Natural remedies, strive to address the cause of a specific ailment through the use of natural processes. In many cases minor alterations in a person's lifestyle helps to eliminate the cause of one's ailment. In other situations use of natural substances can be an effective means to bring the body back to a state of balance.

Some of the most effective and natural alternative remedies for treating High Blood Pressure are given here. In conventional treatments same medicines are given to all persons for same disease but in natural treatments all persons are treated separately depending on their constitution.

A WARNING ABOUT STOPPING DRUGS

> If your doctor has prescribed a blood-pressure lowering drug or combination of drugs for you and you are currently taking them, do not stop all at once or without consulting your doctor.

Chapter 6

Natural methods for treatment of High Blood Pressure

If medicines have side effects how can the blood pressure be reduced and brought under control. Answer to this question lies in change of life style (as advised by above doctors) and change of diet and use of herbs etc.

Treatment by change of life style

The success of your remedy depends on your ability to adjust your lifestyle to reflect what your body positively responds to. For this reason, you should write your Blood Pressure in a diary and also to record your daily routine, changes and observations. Review your diary frequently to see what remedies bring the desired results.

Dr. Kaplan offers this eight-step plan for treating mild hypertension:

1. Weight loss. For the overweight, weight reduction should be the primary goal. The frequency of hypertension is about twice as high in the obese as in the no obese; furthermore, even a small weight loss will often lower the blood pressure. The dual benefits of lowering blood pressure and losing weight should provide incentive to stay on a weight-loss program.
2. Sodium restriction. For all hypertensive, salt in the diet should be restricted to two grams of sodium a day (less than one-half teaspoon). This can be accomplished simply by leaving out salt in cooking and avoiding heavily salted foods such as smoked meats, pickles, and most canned and processed foods. After a few months on a lower sodium diet, the taste preference for salty foods will decrease. However, in order to maintain calcium intake, do not reduce consumption of low-fat, low-sodium milk and cheese products.
3. Fiber/fat in the diet. More high fiber foods and less saturated fat in the diet may also help lower pressure. They are also recommended for cancer immunity and cholesterol reduction.
4. Alcohol. In moderate amounts (less than two ounces a day) alcohol appears to protect against coronary disease. In larger amounts, it may raise blood pressure enough to make it the most prevalent cause of reversible hypertension. Studies suggest that alcohol is responsible for at least 10 percent of hypertension in men and 1

percent of hypertension in women. A reasonable position would be to allow up to, but no more than, two ounces a day.

5. Exercise. After aerobic exercise such as walking, jogging, bicycling, or swimming, blood pressure falls by as much as 25 percent and remains lower for at least 30 minutes.

    CAUTION: However, blood pressure may rise alarmingly during anaerobic exercise such as weight lifting. Regular active exercise of the aerobic type should be encouraged.

6. Potassium. For mild hypertension, potassium supplements are usually not necessary. Potassium intake tends to increase when sodium is reduced, particularly by the substitution of natural foods for canned or processed foods.
7. Other minerals. Magnesium and calcium supplements should only be given to those who are deficient in the minerals until there is more evidence that they produce desired results.
8. Relaxation therapy. Unfortunately, only a few hypertensive will choose to try relaxation therapy, and even fewer will stick with it. Most of those who do will achieve some lowering of blood pressure, and a few will show a considerable decrease. In addition, they may be less anxious and feel better.

Non-drug therapy, following these suggestions may lower the blood pressure to a level below 140/90 for most of the persons with mild hypertension.

Dr. Kaplan tells us, "While the overall expense may be higher, the potential for improvement in overall health makes the cost seem trivial. Whether hypertensive patients take drugs to lower their blood pressure or not, they still need to lose weight, exercise regularly, eat a prudent diet, and learn to relax. Non-drug therapies have a place in the treatment of all hypertensive patients."

As said earlier you should make changes in your life style to prevent high blood pressure. Easiest changes that can be made in life style are

Eat right (eating 5 servings of vegetables and fruits) and reducing the sodium in your diet, exercise more, limit your alcohol intake and lose weight if necessary.

Not only will these four lifestyle changes help you prevent high blood pressure, but they will also keep you safe from a lot of other health problems you could face, from diabetes to cancer.

ADDITIONAL LIFESTYLE TIPS FOR CONTROLLING BLOOD PRESSURE

Get Physically Active

There is no better way to improve the condition of your heart than to exercise it. Getting just a half hour of moderate physical activity at least five days a week can go a long way toward lowering your blood pressure and improving your overall health.
Exercise can help people with high blood pressure no matter what they weigh.
According to a fact sheet provided by the Mayo-Clinic activity is the key to strengthening your heart. And a strong heart pumps more blood with less effort, thus lowering your blood pressure without doing anything else.
Getting more exercise can lower your blood pressure 10 points, and if you do not already have high blood pressure, it can help you prevent it. About 3o minutes of moderate exercise a day is ideal for preventing or reducing high blood pressure (and it will make that weight loss easier, too).

Ideas of moderate aerobic activity:

• Walking, Jogging or Running
• Dancing
• Swimming
• Biking
• Using workout equipment like elliptical trainers, rowing machines, stair step machines, treadmills or ski machines
• Water aerobics

Practice deep breathing techniques. A great way to reduce the tension in a stressful moment is to breathe deeply. Often, when we are stressed out, we start breathing shallowly or even hold our breath. The next time you feel stressed, close your eyes if you can, inhale to a count of six, hold for three seconds and exhale to a count of six. Wait three more seconds and repeat.
Doing this cycle as few as five times, will make you feel lot more in control and help your blood pressure as well.

Do yoga, Tai chi, meditation or other stress-reducing techniques. I am a big fan of yoga because I know that it works to help you feel calm, as well as more flexible, and confident and comfortable in your body--all things that are important for good health. Yoga also includes an emphasis on deep breathing, which is important for relaxation and lowering blood pressure. Tai chi, meditation and other techniques that involve slow, steady movement and deep breathing can also be helpful. Even going for a slow, meditative walk around your neighborhood a couple of times a week can work wonders on your blood pressure.

But there are many other things you can do to prevent high blood pressure or to keep yourself on a healthy road once you have lowered your blood pressure. One of the biggest ones is controlling stress.

Stress Management

Many studies suggest that lowering your stress levels or having a productive way to deal with the stress in your life will keep your blood pressure low. That is one reason aerobic exercises and meditation are helpful Even mild stress can raise your blood pressure, so it is important to have a plan from day to day that will help you reduce stress and deal constructively with the stress you cannot eliminate.

Other things that help to reduce stress include practicing yoga or tai chi, meditation, biofeedback, breathing exercises, and even hypnotherapy. Always take some time away from your busy schedule and focus on relaxation can be helpful. Avoid rushing.

It is important to find a good, productive way to handle your stress. Bottled up stress can raise your blood pressure, heart attacks and other health problems

One other thing that might help you reduce stress and live your optimum life is training your brain to give you its best. You can learn to reduce your stress levels, become more creative, think "smarter" and reduce your sleeping problems.

GET A GOOD NIGHT'S SLEEP

Sleep is vital for reducing stress levels and living a healthy life. If you are not getting enough good quality sleep, it can affect your blood pressure. Getting a good night's sleep is also important for general health and well-being. If you are sleep deprived, you will feel more stress from smaller incidents. These little things that get on your nerves will raise your blood pressure, and could even lead to a heart attack or other health problems.

If you are having trouble sleeping, drinking tea, particularly chamomile, lavender or green tea before bed can be helpful. I have found biochemical medicine KaliPhos very effective in inducing sleep. Setting a sleep schedule will also help you.

Try not to sleep in on the weekends if you can help it, because your body will do better if you keep to a regular sleep schedule. Also, make sure you do not use the bed for anything other than sleeping and sex. If you do work in bed, your mind might associate it as a place for work and stress, which may disturb your sleep. Watching television in bed is a bad idea, too. For one thing, it is stimulation, which you do not need when you are trying to sleep. It also keeps your bedroom from being a relaxing, quiet, peaceful haven, which is what you need if you are looking for a good night's rest.

Getting enough of the right kind of sleep can really improve the quality of your life and give you more energy to do things you love, as well as ridding you of health problems caused by stress over not being able to sleep properly.

Chapter 7

FOOD

Diet plays an important Part in causing/preventing/curing Blood pressure and heart problems. We should avoid saturated fats and take foods that have lot of vitamins and minerals. Biochemical doctors (now all doctors) believe that it is deficiency of minerals that is the root cause of all diseases. (They have 12 medicines,(minerals) only to take care of all types of diseases. It is advised that we take healthy foods to avoid problems.

Eat your vegetables. Getting a varied diet high in vegetables will help you get a lot of the nutrients that are helpful in lowering blood pressure. Aim for four or five servings of vegetables/fruits a day. A great way to add veggies to your diet is to eat a salad for or with your lunch every day. A cup of lettuce with a half-cup of other vegetables added in gives you one serving of vegetables.

Below are given some of the foods that help in preventing/curing B.P, Cholesterols (LDL) and heart problems

Apples: Apples contain a phytochemical called quercetin which acts as a natural anti-inflammatory agent and helps in prevention of blood clots as well. Apples contain vitamins and fiber, which help in maintain good health.

Avocados: Avocados are rich in monounsaturated fats, just like olive oil, plus it is loaded with vitamins and phytochemicals that work as antioxidants to protect your heart (and other parts of your body.
Avocados are also an excellent source of magnesium, fibre and potassium and low in sodium. Eating half an avocado will also add nicely to your daily intake of vitamins C, A, E, and B complex vitamins. The combination of these nutrients and the polyphenols work as antioxidants and make avocados a must-have for any anti-inflammatory diet.

Green leafy vegetables: They are rich in vitamins, minerals and fibre, plus they're low in calories. Eating green leafy vegetables has also been associated with better retention of memory. Use fresh spinach leaves as a salad green or serve Swiss chard or kale as a side dish.

Oats: Oats contain a soluble fiber called beta glucan that helps reduce total and LDL. Soluble fibre also helps keep your digestive system healthy..

Olive oil reduces your risk of B.P and heart problem by lowering your LDL levels.

Salmon, walnuts provide Omega3 that prevents inflammation of heart and veins and help in lowering BP.

Dry beans, such as navy beans, kidney beans, pinto beans and black beans, are an excellent anti-inflammatory source of plant protein, minerals, B complex vitamins and vitamin K. They're also full of beneficial fibre and they contain polyphenols that work as antioxidants. Research suggests dry beans may provide health benefits and help prevent some types of heart disease, diabetes and high blood pressure, as well as reduce inflammation

Krill oil: Krill oil is a very good antioxidant and helps in reducing inflammation and its use will reduce B.P.

Bananas, Broccoli, and Celery – Bananas have been proven to reduce your blood pressure greatly. This is because bananas are rich and high in potassium and through clinical studies has proven to dramatically reduce your blood pressure. Bananas and foods high in potassium can reduce your blood pressure up to 20 points. You can also try other foods that are high in potassium such as avocados, prunes, raisins, and dried apricots.
A high fibre diet has also shown to greatly lower a person's blood pressure. Broccoli is very high in fibre and has been proven to lower your blood pressure also. If you don't particularly like broccoli there are many other foods that you can consume that are high in fibre such as Brussels sprouts, cabbage, carrots, mushrooms, peppers, spinach, and sweet potatoes.
Grapefruits and lemons are also very beneficial in the treatment of high blood pressure. This is because both fruits contain Vitamin P which is effective in preventing capillary fragility and also tones up your arteries.
Indian gooseberry juice and honey can also help you lower your blood pressure when you mix the two ingredients together. Try taking two tablespoons of Indian gooseberry juice and honey mixed together. You can take this mixture every morning on an empty stomach and can be the perfect antidote to naturally lower your blood pressure without the hassle of taking a pill.

Try consuming at least two to three cloves of garlic twice daily. This will not only lower your blood pressure but will also restrict the spasms of small arteries and also moderates your heart beat as well as your pulse rate.

You can also try making a parsley leaf beverage by simmering 20 grams of fresh parsley leaves in 250 ml of water. You can drink this mixture frequently throughout the day and helps improve arterial health.

Using one teaspoon of fenugreek seeds with water each morning on an empty stomach can also maintain and control your blood pressure throughout the day.

You can also mix one teaspoon of cayenne pepper with a half of a cup of lukewarm water daily. This is also a very effective home remedy that will lower your blood pressure dramatically.

It is possible to supplement potassium (though the potassium supplements sold over the counter have very small amounts of potassium and larger doses are only available by prescription), but the best way to get more potassium is through diet. Recent studies have shown that the type of potassium found in most foods is as effective at lowering blood pressure as the type available in supplements.

The recommended daily allowance for potassium is 4,700 milligrams, though most people get much less than that. Even foods that are considered high in potassium do not get you that close to the allowance. Three apricots, for instance, have 314 milligrams, while a banana has about 400.

Here are some foods that are high in potassium:
• Apricots
• Avocado
• Bananas
• Cantaloupe
• Melons
• Kiwi
• Lima beans
• Milk
• Oranges and juice
• Potatoes
• Prunes
• Spinach
• Tomatoes
• Meat, fish, poultry

TOP 10 DIET TIPS FOR HEALTHY BLOOD PRESSURE

Load up on fruit. Fruit, of course, is important for maintaining health. We talked earlier about the importance of vitamin C, which is abundant in citrus fruits. You should also try to get four or five servings of fruit a day. This is hard for a lot of people, but if you work up to it gradually you will find it is not much of a problem. A glass of orange juice at breakfast, a banana (high in potassium!) for a snack and about 16 grapes as an after-dinner treat gets three servings down.

Switch to whole grains. Many of the nutrients that are important for healthy blood pressure are found in whole grains. Oats in particular are helpful for reducing cholesterol, which can also reduce blood pressure. You should try to get at least half of your grains from whole grains.

HOW WHOLE GRAINS HELP CONTROL BLOOD PRESSURE

Whole grains, such as wheat, oats, and millet, are a source of powerful antioxidants that can perform two valuable functions:

- They help bring down excessive blood pressure.
- They help keep readings in a healthful balance.

Whole grains are prime sources of fiber, the substance that is able to push plasma cholesterol levels down, an important factor in blood pressure control. The same fiber releases antioxidants that block absorption of many fatty elements and then break them down for easier elimination.

A bowl of hot oatmeal, for example, with some fruits for natural flavor and sweetening is nourishing and also effective for keeping your pressure in check. It offers both fiber and pectin, a valuable antioxidant that protects against the risk of clots, which are always a threat for the hypertensive. Plan to have this cereal at least three times weekly for good antioxidant fortification, especially in the morning before you start your day's chores.

If you can switch to sprouted grains, they are a stellar source of nutrition. Soaking grains in warm water neutralizes enzyme anti-nutrients (like gluten) present in all grains and stimulates the creation of numerous beneficial enzymes for easy digestion.
The action of these good enzymes also increases the amount of many vitamins, especially B vitamins.
Eating a moderate amount of properly soaked, sprouted and sourdough fermented grains can be part of a good diet, even if you are gluten sensitive.

All grains and seeds can be sprouted following these basic instructions though the germination time may vary from grain to grain. Take care to choose only organic, untreated grains as they tend to sprout more evenly and reliably.

Choose clean grains and rinse thoroughly. In a ceramic or steel crock, pour enough warm water over grains until they are submerged in a couple inches of water. Soak overnight. Rinse and stir the grains a couple times during the next day. Repeat process for 2-3 days until sprouted. To make flour, rinse, drain and refrigerate or dehydrate before grinding.

Eat fish. Two or three servings of fish weekly are a great way to protect your heart, and the fish oil can reduce high blood pressure. If you do not eat fish, supplement with fish oil capsules or one tablespoon of flaxseed oil daily.

Make it lean. Go for lean meats and poultry whenever possible. Lower-fat meats, including fish, are always a healthy choice. Also consider lower-fat dairy products and even including some soy in your diet, if you do not already.

Nuts. Nuts are a great snack, and many nuts are filled with micronutrients and vitamins that can keep you healthy. They may reduce the risk of heart disease, help you keep a healthy weight and reduce your risk of diabetes. An ounce of walnuts daily gives you all the Omega 3s you need, while almonds are a great source of vitamin E. Brazil nuts are a great source of potassium and selenium.

Drink more water. Hydration is important for all sorts of reasons, but a wonderful benefit that comes from drinking enough water is cleaning out any waste that has accumulated in the body. Drinking water will help flush out sodium, in addition to other waste products in the body. Drinking lots of water helps you feel more full, which is helpful when trying to lose weight. Water helps your body function at its peak.

Try substituting one caloric beverage a day for water until you are drinking at least eight glasses a day.

Pass on the refined salts. Though the link between high-sodium diets and high blood pressure is not conclusive, many people with high blood pressure are sensitive to the sodium in salt--especially refined salts. Most people get way more salt than they need. Try using seas salts or seasoning with other spices that bring more flavours to dishes you cook at home. Cut down on prepared or pre-packaged foods, which are filled with more salt than anyone needs.

Eat more organics. Organic foods are grown and processed without the use of pesticides and other man-made chemicals. They are thought to include more healthy nutrients than conventionally produced foods, and their production is less stressful to the planet. Organics can be expensive, so start transferring to organics gradually or only buy organic varieties of foods that typically have the highest pesticide load, such as peaches, strawberries, bell peppers, apples and lettuce.

Drink green tea. It reduces blood pressure and improves heart health. Green tea contains more of the healthful compounds. Drink at least one cup of tea daily, hot or cold, and you will see all sorts of health benefits. Cut out one soda or cup of coffee a day and drink GREEN tea instead.

Chapter 8

Electrolytes and B.P

Importance of salt and other electrolytes in control of B.P

It is said the small amounts of salt can cause elevation in pressure with serious repercussions. Salt destroys antioxidants weakening the immune system. To protect against high blood pressure, limit or eliminate the use of salt in all forms. This is true especially for persons who are sensitive to salt but does not apply to all persons.

Cutting consumption of salt and sodium can help many people to control hypertension. This is especially true for blacks and older persons as they are more sensitive to salt. Genetic plays a big role in sensitivity of salt.

In experiments made in 32 countries, the results revealed few links between salt intake and hypertension in people. Howsoever in countries that had extremely high intake of salt, tended to have higher level of B.P, while individuals with very little intake of salt in their diet had lower levels. But these are the extremes. For most people in most countries, there was little association between salt and sodium consumption and B.P. With persons having normal B.P if the consumption of salt is increased excessively, the B.P will go up but on reduction of salt, the B.P will come back. Findings suggest that except in abnormal conditions, salt consumption does not increase B.P

In another research 841 men and women were observed the effect of diet on B.P. Some persons lowered calories, some salt and other both. Group that reduced calories were found to have the highest lowering of B.P while group who controlled salt were least affected in lowering of B.P.

Mild effects of dietary salt restriction on BP hardly seem worth the effort. But these results do not rule out the possibility that an individual patient occasionally will have a more substantial response to salt restriction. This is mostly applicable to persons having overweight, older and hypertensive as these persons are more salt sensitive.

To know whether restricting your salt will lower your B.P, experiment by measuring your B.P for a few days after cutting your salt intake and observe if reduction of Salt in all forms reduces your B.P or not.

In case you find that you are sensitive to salt/sodium intake you should eliminate salt from your diet, but at the same time, you need to boost your intake of other electrolytes like potassium, calcium and magnesium.

One study showed that 9 out of 20 elderly hypertensive patients experienced an 11 point drop in their daytime systolic blood after substituting table salt with potassium, magnesium, calcium. It is the balancing act of all these electrolytes that helps in reducing B.P. These minerals have an antioxidant reaction that washes out the molecular fragments to help control pressure. Potassium plays an important role in energy release from foods to maintain a normal flow of nerve signals and muscle contractions.

If you are taking prescription diuretics to wash out sodium from your system, they may also wash out needed potassium (both seem to exist simultaneously in most foods).
This could cause diarrhea, nausea, and severe malnutrition.
To protect against such disorders, plan to minimize salt intake and also to include more potassium foods in your menu program.

Unless you are sodium-sensitive, chances are your high blood pressure stems from a lack of the correct proportions of calcium, magnesium and potassium.

The fact is your body needs sodium as an essential nutrient and your body cannot produce its own sodium.

Natural chloride increases your body's ability to absorb heart healthy potassium.
Chloride is the key for balanced stomach acidity, helps sustain healthy pH for the whole body and increases the elimination of CO_2 from your blood, preventing acidosis.
It turns out that natural sea salt — rich in natural potassium, magnesium and sodium — helps to normalize healthy blood pressure levels.
On the other hand, unnatural, isolated, synthetic sodium chloride (table salt) is a different story. Table salt has ZERO trace elements and, because your body cannot use it, the synthetic salt becomes a biological poison. Basically, standard table salt has lost its essential qualities when it is manufactured and refined.

When you add pinch of genuine sea salt to a glass of water and drink it, you are releasing and activating powerful, ion-charged minerals and trace elements. Without these, your body cannot produce electricity and slowly drowns in its own CO_2, in a slow death caused by a severe pH imbalance called "acidosis".

One of the first symptoms of acidosis, or severe acid pH, is high blood pressure. High blood pressure symptoms can also be triggered from dehydration, so it is crucial that you help balance healthy blood pressure levels with natural sea salt intake along with plenty of water.

Table salt is slightly more than 40 percent sodium.
• One teaspoon of table salt (5 g) contains 2,200 mg of sodium.
• The average person daily consumes 2 teaspoons to 4 teaspoons of salt, or 4,400 mg to 8,800 mg of sodium.
• Allowing for individual differences, the recommended daily allowance for sodium is 1,100 mg to 3,300 mg for adults (1/2 teaspoon to 1'/2 teaspoons of salt) daily.
Enough sodium is obtained from natural foods and water for your basic needs so you need not be concerned about your daily needs. But if you must have salt in your meal plan, then limit yourself to about 1 teaspoon daily.

Here are some ways to enjoy natural flavors without salt:

• Use lemon and lime wedges on many foods. These tart fruits are almost sodium-free. You'll enjoy a fragrant, tangy flavor that makes up for the absence of salt.
• Avoid salt in cooking or at your table. Switch to flavorful natural herbs and spices.
• Salt-free butter and margarine are available.
• Many canned, frozen, dehydrated, and processed foods and beverages are high in sodium. Read labels. Select salt-free brands.
• Many prepackaged breakfast foods are high in sodium; others are low. Again, read labels and make a wise choice.
• Homemade salad dressings (oil-vinegar-herbs) contain little sodium. Commercial dressings and mayonnaise (unless otherwise labeled) are high in sodium.
• Most fresh meats and poultry products are low in sodium, but processed meats (ham, bacon, sausage, frankfurters, etc.) are high in this pressure-raising flavoring.
• Fresh fish is rather low in sodium, but processed fish often has added salt. The label tells all.

A few extra moments spent in food selection and preparation can add years to your life by restoring a sparkling clean cardiovascular system and a healthy blood pressure.

Below is Sodium-Potassium-Calorie Counter to help you maintain proper sodium potassium ratio.

Vegetables*	Portion	Sodium (mg.)	Potassium (mg.)	Calories
Peas				
Fresh	2/3 cup	1	196	71
Canned	3/4 cup	236	96	88
Potatoes				
Boiled (in skin)				
medium		3	407	76
French Fried				
10 pieces		3	427	137
Radishes	10 small	18	322	17
Sauerkraut	2/3 cup	747	140	18
Spinach	1/2 cup	45	291	21
Tomatoes				
Raw	1 medium	4	366	33
Canned	V2 cup	130	217	21
Paste	312 oz.	38	888	82

*Note: Because vegetable counts vary greatly from raw to cooked state, values are for cooked vegetables with no added salt unless otherwise noted.

Frozen vegetables have virtually the same count as fresh vegetables, when cooked, unless otherwise noted.

PRESSURE-RAISING COMPOUNDS TO AVOID

 To protect against raising B.P, you would do well to avoid these pressure-raising substances.

Remember, read labels before you use any product to see if it contains these destructive salts.

1. Salt (sodium chloride)—whether in cooking or at the table, salt should be avoided. Salt is also found in processed foods unless otherwise noted.

2. Baking powder—used to leaven quick breads and cakes, sometimes added to cooking vegetables or used as an alkalizer for indigestion problems. Its sodium contributes to high blood pressure, heart disease, and kidney problems. It releases carbon dioxide gas into the digestive organs which can be painful and dangerous.

4. Brine (table salt and water)—used in processing foods to inhibit growth of bacteria; in cleaning or blanching fruits and vegetables; in freezing and canning certain foods; and for flavor as in corned beef, pickles, and sauerkraut.

5. Disodium phosphate—found in quick-cooking cereals and processed Cheeses.

6. Monosodium glutamate—sold under various brand names for home use as a flavor-enhancer; also in many packaged, canned, and frozen foods.

7. Sodium alginate—used in many chocolate milks and ice creams for smooth texture.

8. Sodium benzoate—used as a preservative in many condiments, such as relishes, sauces, and salad dressings.

9. Sodium hydroxide—used in food processing to soften and loosen skins of ripe olives, hominy, and some fruits and vegetables, also used in preparing so-called Dutch process cocoa and chocolate.

10. Sodium propionate—used in pasteurized cheeses and some commercially baked goods to inhibit mold.

11. Sodium sulfite—used to bleach certain fruits for artificial color, such as maraschino cherries and glazed or crystallized fruit; also used as a preservative in some dried fruit. Read labels.

(TIP: Select naturally sun-dried fruits.)

If you must use packaged or prepared foods and beverages, read labels. In case of presence of sodium in any form you should avoid the product. In so doing, you will protect your arterial walls against erosion. And you will give "breathing space" to your antioxidants so they will build resistance to the threat of high blood pressure.

Calcium, Magnesium and Potassium play a very vital role in control of Blood Pressure.

It is possible to supplement potassium (though the potassium supplements sold over the counter have very small amounts of potassium and larger doses are only available by prescription), but the best way to get more potassium is through diet. Recent studies have shown that the type of potassium found in most foods is as effective at lowering blood pressure as the type available in supplements.

The recommended daily allowance for potassium is 4,700 milligrams, though most people get much less than that. Even foods that are considered high in potassium do not get you that close to the allowance. Three apricots, for instance, have 314 milligrams, while a banana has about 400.

Here are some foods that are high in potassium:
• Apricots
• Avocado
• Bananas
• Cantaloupe
• Melons
• Kiwi
• Lima beans
• Milk
• Oranges and juice
• Potatoes
• Prunes
• Spinach
• Tomatoes
• Meat, fish, poultry

MARVELOUS MAGNESIUM

Magnesium is a micronutrient found in the bones, body tissues and organs of the body.
It is necessary for normal muscle and nerve function, steady heartbeat, strong bones and a healthy immune system. Potassium and magnesium actually work together in the body, so if you have low magnesium levels, it is likely your potassium levels will be low as well.

It is recommended that most people get around 400 milligrams of magnesium a day. Again, taking diuretics may flush magnesium from your body, so supplementation or eating extra foods rich in magnesium may be necessary.

There is not as much evidence regarding magnesium's effectiveness in treating high blood pressure as there is for potassium, but the DASH diet calls for 500 milligrams of magnesium daily and many studies suggest that a combination of potassium, magnesium (and often calcium) and fibre are protective of the heart and can reduce high blood pressure. It is relatively easy to get your daily dose of magnesium. A cup of black beans, for example, has 120 milligrams and two ounces of almonds have 156 milligrams.

Foods that are high in magnesium include:
• Whole-grain bread
• Dark green leafy vegetables
• Halibut
• Most kinds of nuts, especially almonds and cashews
• Soybeans
• Oatmeal
• Potatoes
• Peanut butter
• Black-eyed peas
• Yogurt

CONSIDER CALCIUM

Calcium is the third member of the nutrient trio that is often mentioned as important for the reduction of high blood pressure. Most people know that calcium helps keep the bones and teeth healthy, but it is also essential for the proper functioning of muscles and nerves and helps blood clot.

There is no consensus as to whether calcium supplementation is helpful for reducing high blood pressure, but, again, it was one of the nutrients that the DASH study focused on. It recommends 1,250 milligrams a day, while the RDA is 1,000 milligrams for most adults. Eight ounces of calcium-fortified orange juice gets you 250 milligrams, while a cup of reduced or non-fat milk has 300 milligrams.

Even if calcium does not lower high blood pressure, most studies agree that having low levels of calcium can raise blood pressure. So it is important to try to get the recommended amount of calcium, whether through supplements or diet.

The following foods are good natural sources of Calcium:

• Broccoli
• Dairy products (preferably low-fat)
• Salmon
• Spinach

- Tofu
- Orange juice
- Cereal and other foods fortified with calcium

Chapter 9

Effect of Molecular Wastes/Free Radicals on blood pressure

An accumulation of free radicals can destroy healthy cells that make up your arteries and arterioles. Ordinary blood pressure can be withstood by these pipelines of your cardio-vascular system. But the molecular wastes and radicals cause erosion of your vein and artery walls. The molecular discards, or frees radicals also cause blockages in the arteries increasing pressure required for pumping of blood and increasing the risk of cardiovascular distress.

To have proper BP, it is important that these free radicals should be removed by antioxidants. This can be achieved by changing your diet. You should adopt fresh juices, raw foods (vegetables and fruits.).It is said that you should take at least 5 servings of these vegetables and fruits daily for good health.

This spares your digestive system to metabolize heavier foods. Your antioxidants are free to work solely upon raw foods, using the nutrients in them to help remove the harmful free radicals. This helps strengthen your cardiovascular system and ease the destruction of arteries.

Once the harmful radicals have been detoxified from your system, your blood moves better through your arteries and veins and your blood pressure tends to level off.

Garlic is highly antioxidant that resists the attack of radicals. Garlic and even onions can be used as anti-oxidants.

Garlic uses process called mitogenetic to regulate blood pressure almost immediately. It has an accelerated effect because of the detoxification power of the mitogenetic reaction that synthesizes and breaks down of lipids in liver and washing out the wastes responsible for clogging. Specifically, garlic has a dilating effect on the blood vessels, allowing better circulation and transport of nutrients. Garlic also removes symptoms such as angina-like pain, dizziness, and head. Asians have used garlic to lower pressure for many centuries.

A combination of onions and garlic, two powerful antioxidant foods, can work miracles in helping you achieve a healthy blood pressure. Their antioxidant detoxification works even better when used together.

Onions are a prime source of antioxidants that removes thromboxane, a poisonous free radical that causes blood pressure to soar. Antioxidants of onions work against platelet aggregation, which can trigger off dangerously high blood pressure.

Garlic is a prime source of selenium (the valuable antioxidant needed to normalize pressure), which also prevents cellular adhesion and clot formation.

A combination of both of these antioxidants initiates an action that gives natural immunity to the risk of high blood pressure.

Both onions and garlic release antioxidants that inhibit the treacherous buildup of wastes that raise blood pressure.

Plan to use this combination on a daily basis for the sake of your pressure and your life.

There are case studies where use of Garlic and onion reduced high blood pressure within two days.

All Natural Antioxidant Health Tonic.

If you hate scent of onions and/or garlic, you can enjoy their benefits when used as a tasty tonic.

In a glass of fresh salt-free vegetable juice, place several slices of fresh onion and three or four garlic cloves. Blenderize until frothy for two or three minutes, then sip slowly. You have a tangy and tasty treat that is not only a thirst quencher, but is also a richly concentrated source of biologically active antioxidants. Within moments, the selenium and allicin components will be building immunity to the risk of high blood pressure.

Just one glass a day of this "All-Natural Antioxidant Health Tonic" increases immunity to the risks of hypertension and cardiovascular distress.

There are case histories where High B.P was brought under control within 2 days by using Garlic and onion and within 3 days with health tonic.

Some other natural antioxidants

Cocoa bean extract can support healthy cholesterol levels. A study in The American Journal of Clinical Nutrition found that supplementing with cocoa powder and dark chocolate may help reduce LDL cholesterol and reduce B.P.

Researchers attribute this effect to Substances known as flavan-3-oils found in cocoa products. This is important. Because when that bad cholesterol mixes with free radicals, it oxidizes free radicls inside the arteries. A recent study published in the Archives of Internal Medicine found that eating or drinking cocoa lowered blood pressure and reduced the risk of death in older men.

Men who ate chocolate regularly, over a 15-year study, were found to have lower blood pressure than those who did not, even when weight, smoking, physical activity and other factors were taken into account.

Pomegranate extract also protects against free radicals and oxidative stress helping to support healthy cholesterol and B.P. But instead of having to drink a sugary juice every day, you can slip in the benefits along with the other VitaCardio nutrients.

Chapter 10

AYUERVEDA AND BLOOD PRESSURE

Ayurvedic medicine is a discipline of medicine that originated in India. It suggests that different people have different body types and therefore have to be treated in different ways when it comes to healing diseases.

Unless you know about Ayurvedic medicine, you should not attempt to treat yourself. A knowledgeable practitioner can tell you what herbs, and in what doses, are going to be most beneficial for you. Some of the most popular Ayurvedic remedies for high blood pressure include sankhapuspi, ashwagandha, garlic, valerian, gotu kola and trikatu, and Ginseng besides others.

Ginseng is a rather controversial blood pressure remedy because some people say that it helps lower blood pressure, while others say it helps raise blood pressure. The theory is that ginseng is generally a blood pressure moderator, and whether your blood pressure is high or low, it will help you get it to a more normal level.

In a Korean study in which people took 1.5 grams of red Asian ginseng three times a day for eight weeks, participants reduced their blood pressure by about five percent. This study is interesting because it studied people with what is known as "white coat hypertension," that is, people who have a spike in blood pressure just going to the doctor. It is possible the ginseng reduced their stress levels rather than acting directly on blood pressure, but either way it was helpful.

Drinking as little as a half cup a day of green or oolong tea for a year could cut the risk of hypertension by as much as 50 percent, according to a study done in Taiwan.

Arjuna is another strong herb that helps in controlling LDL and Blood pressure.

Breaking research from top institutions shows that this "warrior" extract doesn't just support healthy blood pressure. It may help

- Maintain healthy circulation—both vital for a powerful cardiovascular system and a full, active life.

- Keep cholesterol in the healthy range — so you and your family can rest easy at night.

- Promote endothelial cell function — these are the cells that line and protect your blood vessels.

In fact, a 2007 animal study at the Bose Institute showed that this extract helped boost antioxidant activity, reduced damage from free radicals, and could be an all-around cardio protector.

The warrior (Arjuna) extract might be the most important natural breakthrough in heart health — ever. And the studies keep stacking up, showing that it may also help…

- Support heart function during exertion and exercise — when you need it most.

- Fight damage caused by free radicals — so you can enjoy youthful energy and stamina for years to come.

- Strengthen your most important muscle — so you can get out and play with your grandkids or make it through all 18 holes

- It's a powerful antioxidant. Like the warrior Arjuna vanquished his enemies on the battlefield…Arjuna extract can help defeat the free radicals that can age your heart. Didn't lead the healthiest life in the past? It's never too late to take a step in the right direction.

- It also has a relaxing effect on blood vessels. For people who are concerned with blood pressure, Arjuna may help keep it in the healthy range. So you relax and rest easy knowing you've got the support you need in any situation.

- Dr. Alan Keith Tillotson, in his book One Earth Herbal Sourcebook, says Arjuna is especially helpful in promoting a healthy inflammation response. Inflammation is an important part of your body's natural defenses. But it is critical for your good health to keep it in just the right balance.

- It can help keep blood flowing smooth and steady to and from the heart. (And men, when blood flows strong it can have a powerful effect on your other most important organ…)

- Arjuna naturally contains Coq10—a chemical your body needs to provide energy to your entire body. Your heart requires the most energy…and Arjuna helps make sure you're getting it.

Arjuna may help support heart function during exercise, too. 1,500 mg of Arjuna helped one group of people add an average of six more minutes to their treadmill time. They recovered easier too. So you can lead your active lifestyle without worry.

CHAPTER 11

The High Blood Pressure Natural Remedies

Garlic is probably one of the most popular herbal supplements out there. Garlic is a bulb that is popularly used for flavoring in cooking, but it is also beneficial for the heart and is known to help lower cholesterol.

The volatile compounds in garlic — especially allicin, which is what gives garlic its pungent smell — are thought to be beneficial for lowering blood pressure and cholesterol levels.

Garlic supplements should provide at least 10 milligrams of allicin in a daily dose. Commission E, which sets guidelines for dietary supplements and herbs in Germany, suggests that garlic supplements should provide the equivalent of 4,000 milligrams of fresh garlic--somewhere between one and four cloves depending on the size.

This amount of garlic (or commercial garlic preparation) consumed daily can lower systolic blood pressure five to eleven points and diastolic pressure up to five points. The reduction in blood pressure is most significant when real, whole garlic is eaten, but the garlic supplements are also effective and better than nothing if you do not like to eat garlic.

COENZYME Q10

Coenzyme Q10, known as CoQio for short, is a supplement use of which is growing among people with many health problems.

CoQio is produced by the body and is needed for the basic functioning of cells. Levels of CoQio are thought to decrease as people get older, and are often lower than normal in people with health conditions like heart disease, cancer, diabetes and other ailments.

In fact, in some studies, nearly 40 percent of people with high blood pressure had low levels of CoQio, which strongly suggests that supplementing CoQio is helpful for those with high blood pressure.

CoQio has been used to treat everything from arthritis to Alzheimer's, to boost exercise performance among healthy people and to lower blood pressure. According to the Mayo Clinic, using CoQio is most effective as a treatment for high blood pressure. Small drops in blood pressure have been seen after several weeks of use. The standard dose is around loo milligrams daily.

Hawthorn is an herb widely used in Europe to treat cardiovascular problems. Both the berries and the flowers of the hawthorn plant are used in herbal preparations to make the heart and cardiovascular systems more efficient.

Hawthorn widens the blood vessels, so it works in a similar way to the conventional ACE inhibitor drugs. Its ability to lower blood pressure is rather mild compared to some of the other supplements you could be taking, but it is also thought to generally improve the condition of the heart when taken for several weeks.

The recommended dose for hawthorn is 100 to 250 milligrams of hawthorn preparation with 10 percent procyanidins (the active ingredient in hawthorn) three times a day. You may have to take it for up to a month before you see effects.

TAKE YOUR VITAMINS

Many vitamins have been shown to have an effect on blood pressure, particularly vitamins C, E, B5, B6 and folic acid, which is also a B vitamin.

Folic acid, found in green leafy vegetables and many enriched food products (because it prevents birth defects), reduces homocysteine levels in the blood. Homocysteine is a risk factor for heart disease, and higher levels leave you at higher risk for heart problems.

Young women who consumed at least one milligram of folic acid daily had a 46 percent lower risk of high blood pressure than those who consumed less, while older women had an 18 percent reduced incidence of high blood pressure. The recommended dose for folic acid is 400 micrograms a day.

Vitamin B6 also affects homocysteine levels and is vital for metabolism. It is found in beans, meat, poultry and fortified cereals, as well as some fruits and vegetables. The recommended amount of B6 varies, but it is less than two milligrams for most people.

One study gave participants five milligrams per day per two pounds of body weight and significantly reduced blood pressure in just four weeks, with an average drop of about 10 points each for both systolic and diastolic pressure.

Vitamin B5, which comes from beans, peas, vegetables, fish and whole grains, helps the body make coenzyme A, a deficiency of which can cause low energy levels. It may help improve heart function and detoxify the body. There are no supplements of coenzyme A; it has to be made by the body.

Supplements that claim to be coenzyme A are really B5, calcium, magnesium and other nutrients, so you might as well save your money and eat a diet rich in these other nutrients.

A 500-milligram supplement of vitamin C was found to reduce blood pressure by about nine percent. That is much higher than the recommended daily amount of 60 milligrams a day, but it is safe to take vitamin C in high doses. The thought is that vitamin C protects the body's levels of nitric oxide, a compound that dilates the blood vessels and helps to lower blood pressure. Since vitamin C is an antioxidant, it may help protect the body's level of nitric oxide when it is under stress.

Vitamin E is generally thought to be very helpful for the heart. It can help break down blood clots, improve circulation and strengthen the heartbeat. Vitamin E is recommended to people with high blood pressure more for these reasons more than for significantly lowering blood pressure.

Since high blood pressure is a risk factor in other heart problems, it makes sense to supplement vitamin E to prevent further damage. The RDA is 10 milligrams a day, but it is safe to take much more. Nuts, wheat, apples and dark greens are good sources of vitamin E. If you want to supplement, buy the natural vitamin E pills made with dalpha-tocopherol, which is easier for your body to work with.

OTHER POTENTIALLY HELPFUL SUPPLEMENTS AND ALTERNATIVE OPTIONS

Selenium

Along with zinc and copper, selenium may be helpful for people with high blood pressure. These three nutrients are often low in people with heart disease, so it makes sense that supplementing them may be helpful to people with heart problems or high blood pressure.

You can probably get enough of all three of these nutrients by taking a good quality multivitamin. Selenium comes from meat, dark greens, wheat, walnuts and Brazil nuts.

Zinc can be found in meat, dairy, and beans. Copper is in seafood, nuts, legumes and leafy dark greens.

Beta glucan

Beta glucan is found in oat bran and maltase mushrooms. It is beneficial for lowering cholesterol, which can help lower blood pressure if you already have high cholesterol.

Oat bran is particularly helpful for moving waste materials out of the body. Around 200 milligrams, or about a teaspoon, of oat bran daily can help lower cholesterol and may be beneficial for high blood pressure.

L-Arginine

An amino acid that helps the body produce nitric acid, L-arginine may be helpful in lowering blood pressure. It can be found in meat, peanuts, soy and wheat products. A study that involved taking two grams of L-arginine daily found that participants reduced systolic pressure 20 points after taking the supplement for just a few days. L-arginine is also helpful for lowering cholesterol.

Lecithin

Lecithin helps the body eliminate fat and can help improve liver function. Its function in the body is similar to the Omega 3 fatty acids. (See more on Omega 3 fatty acids below.)

One good source for lecithin is beef and sheep brains, but the supplements you will find in the market are made from soy. Another good source is egg yolks. The main problem with supplementing with lecithin is that it tastes awful. You can buy it in capsules but to get the recommended dose of around three tablespoons a day, you would be taking most of an expensive bottle of pills daily. The granules are much cheaper but unpleasant to eat.

You can make them a little more palatable by eating them off a spoon coated with molasses and washing the dose down with milk. You can also mix them into a cold beverage, although the granules will not dissolve in the liquid.

Fish Oil

Fish oil, also known as Omega 3 fatty acid, is very helpful for the heart. If you eat fish two or three times a week, which many nutritional guidelines recommend, you are probably getting enough fish oil to protect your heart and lower your blood pressure.

If not, supplementation may be in order. There are many high quality fish oil supplements out there, but there are also a lot that are not as good or do not include the amount of fatty acids the label suggests. If possible, ask your doctor, pharmacist or a natural health expert for a recommendation of a good brand.

If you do not eat fish because you are a vegetarian, you can also supplement with flaxseed oil. Flax contains alpha-linoleic acid, another term for Omega 3s, and is often more cost-effective than taking as many as 10 fish oil capsules a day.

Studies have shown that consuming just a tablespoon of flaxseed oil daily may lower both blood pressure numbers by about nine points. Some studies have shown that fish oil oxidizes very easily and thus should be taken with a vitamin E supplement so the body is better able to use it. If you are already taking E for your heart, taking fish oil at the same time will give you the benefits of both.

Apple Cider Vinegar

Many people have had success treating high blood pressure with apple cider vinegar, perhaps because it is high in so many of the vitamins and nutrients that are thought to be helpful in lowering high blood pressure.

Apple cider vinegar includes vitamins C, A, E, Bi, B2 and B6, in addition to potassium, magnesium, copper and many other helpful nutrients. Being vinegar, it does not taste great, but a common way to take it is to mix two tablespoons in eight ounces of water and add some honey to taste. Some people also throw in a garlic clove for even more heart-healthy benefits.

The usefulness of apple cider vinegar for high blood pressure is largely anecdotal, that is, there have not been any studies showing its effectiveness. Still, given what is in it, it makes sense that it would help.

Mix 1 Tablespoon of ACV in 8oz of water.

- Drink 2 to 3 times a day – slowly.

Alternatively- Mix 1 Tablespoon of ACV + ¼ teaspoon baking soda in 8oz of water.

- Drink 2 to 3 times a day – slowly.

Cayenne Pepper

Cayenne is another herb that is thought to benefit the heart in all sorts of ways. It improves circulation and keeps the arteries from hardening.

Proponents of cayenne (actually capsicum, the component that makes hot peppers hot) say it is one of the best things you can take to help your heart, and some claim it can actually stop a heart attack.

Mix a teaspoon of cayenne into a glass of water and drink twice a day. Some people can work up to a tablespoon a glass, but you need to do it gradually to get your body used to it. Some people prefer to take it in hot water seasoned with lemon or honey.

Hot peppers like habaneros, cayenne and jalapenos contain a variety of capsaicinoids, the compounds that give peppers their characteristic heat.

One of the capsaicinoids—capsaicin—is already highly revered in holistic medicine and used to help boost the metabolism and promote weight loss, manage psoriasis, reduce pain, and ease digestive disorders.

And both holistic and conventional medical practitioners use of capsaicin in creams to relieve even the worst arthritis.

That's because capsaicinoids block the action of the enzyme-cyclooxygenase-2. You might know it better as COX-2.

What those doctors don't usually know is why that's important to your blood pressure. It turns out that COX-2 causes the blood vessels to restrict and contract, and this reduces blood flow to the heart and the rest of the body. Reduced blood flow forces your heart to pump harder, which ultimately leads to increased blood pressure. By blocking COX-2, capsaicin lowers blood pressure.

And the capsaicin in hot peppers also has the extraordinary ability to enhance your heart's performance while lowering blood pressure by "capsaicin receptors."

Summary of Remedies for treatment of High Blood Pressure

1. ACV
Mix 1 Tablespoon of ACV in 8oz of water.
- Drink 2 to 3 times a day – slowly.
Alternatively
Mix 1 Tablespoon of ACV with ¼ teaspoon baking soda in 8oz of water.
- Drink 2 to 3 times a day – slowly.

2. Potassium
The Remedy: - Eat fruits and vegetables with at least 350mg per serving at each meal.
- The recommended daily potassium is 4,700 mg.

3. **Magnesium**

The Remedy: - 500-1000 mg twice, daily.
- 250 to 500 mg magnesium taken in the morning and evening.

4. **Omega-3**

The Remedy: - Eat fish 2-3 times a week. OR
1 table spoon of flaxseed oil (obtained through cold pressing of seeds) daily.
1 to 2 tablespoons ground flaxseed (add to cereal, yoghurt, smoothie)

5. **Calcium**
   The Remedy: - 1,250mg is recommended daily.

6. **Garlic**
   The Remedy: - Take one clove of raw garlic each morning.

7. **CoQ10**
   The Remedy: - 100mg per day.

8. **Vitamin C**
   The Remedy: - 500mg per day of Vitamin C (L –ascorbate acid, not L-ascorbic acid).

9. **Cayenne Pepper**
   The Remedy: - 1 teaspoon per day. Add to your morning tea, soups or other foods.
   It can even be added to your ACV drink for an extra kick.

CHAPTER 12

Other natural methods

Yogasana

Yogasana helps in controlling stress and reduces Blood pressure.

To decrease mental tension and regain inner peace, resort to Pranayama, Vipashyna, Transcendental Meditation or Biofeedback. Yoga asanas are extremely beneficial to patients of high blood pressure. Dr.Udupa of Banaras Hindu University's Institute of Medical Sciences tried selected yoga asanas (especially Shavasana) on 25 patients, whose high blood pressure could not be brought down by other means. These patients were continuously monitored and their blood and urine samples periodically examined. Laboratory investigations resorted to, included plasma cholamine level, plasma cortisol level and urinary V. M. A. level. At the end of three months, there was a notable reduction in all these three factors, besides the blood pressure. The results have been tabulated below:

No.	Investigation	Before treatment	After treatment
1	Blood pressure	152/102	139/90
2	Plasma catecholamine	289.82	234.91
3	Plasma cortisol	27.49	25.02
4	Urinary VMA	2.48	2.05

Dr. Udupa considers Shavasana to be extremely beneficial in high blood pressure. Besides, other asanas like Padmasana, Vajrasana, Yogamudra, Dhanurasana, Paschimottanasana, Konasana, Matsyasana and Matsyendrasana should be learnt from a good teacher or a good book and practised regularly.

All such asanas in which the body is held upside down (e.g., Sarvangasana, Shirshasana) are prohibited in high blood pressure.

Magnetic treatment for high Blood pressure

Give Magnet Therapy a chance: It has been seen that many a person with high blood pressure are benefitted by Magnet Therapy.

Magnetic treatment

(1) The magnetic wrist belt should be continuously worn on the right wrist. This belt consists of both the poles. Even North Pole can be used on wrist. The blood pressure gradually comes down.

(2) The south pole of a weak magnet should be applied to the forehead for 5-30 Minutes, 2-3 times a day.

(3) The north pole of a small magnet should be stuck to the web between the great toe and the first toe of the foot.

(4) Magnetised water should be drunk. To magnetise water it is kept in a bottle on a strong magnet.

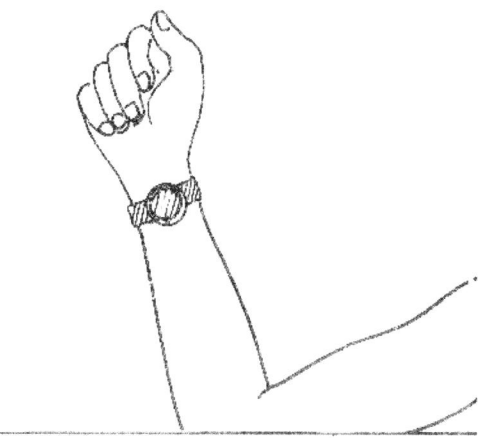

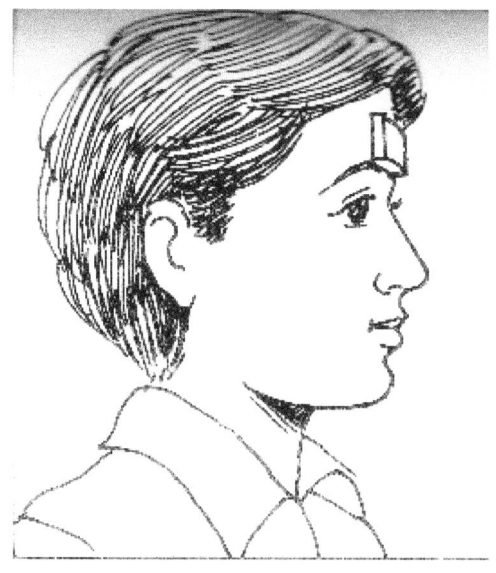

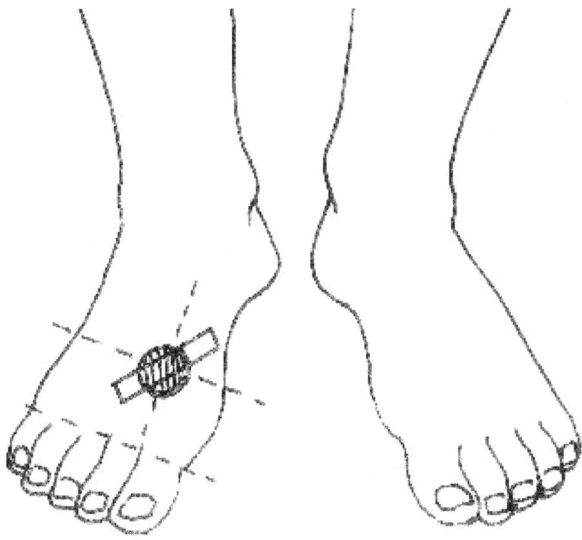

Dr. R. S. Thacker of Delhi advises that the treatment of high blood pressure should be carried out by Method I, namely by applying magnets in both hands, but care should be taken to see that strong magnets are not applied to such persons for long periods. Treatment for five minutes in such cases may be sufficient. He feels that the magnet increases heat in the body.

In high blood pressure, there is already heat and rush of blood to head. He, therefore, advises that a wet towel folded into several layers should be put on the lower part of the spine and it will quickly afford relief to the patient, as that portion of the spine is directly connected with the head.

In the case of low blood pressure, he places two magnets in the hands of the patients, for 10 minutes or even longer and also applies a strong magnet on the lower part of the spine of such patients. Dr.Thacker's method of applying three magnets at a time corresponds to the method adopted by Dr. Mesmer, although for a different disease. Dr. Thacker sometimes applies even more than three magnets to a patient at the same time, if necessary.

Acupressure treatment for high Blood pressure

Good results have been obtained by Acupressure treatment, in mild or moderate blood pressure.

The systolic blood pressure comes down rapidly after initiating Acupressure treatment but the diastolic pressure comes down gradually. Acupressure has enabled quite a few patients to cut down the dosage of antihypertensive drugs by 33 to 50 per cent. This is also a big gain.

The following Acupressure points should be used:

(1) The point located on the middle of a vertical line joining the two ears after they have been folded.

(2) The point located on the outer end of the elbow crease formed due to bending of the elbow.

(3) The point located four fingerbreadths above the inner prominence of the ankle bone and slightly to the backside

(4) The point located four fingerbreadths below the lower margin of the round knee-bone and slightly to the outer dope side, after the knee has been bent at a right angle.

(5) The point located in the flesh between the first (big) and the second toes

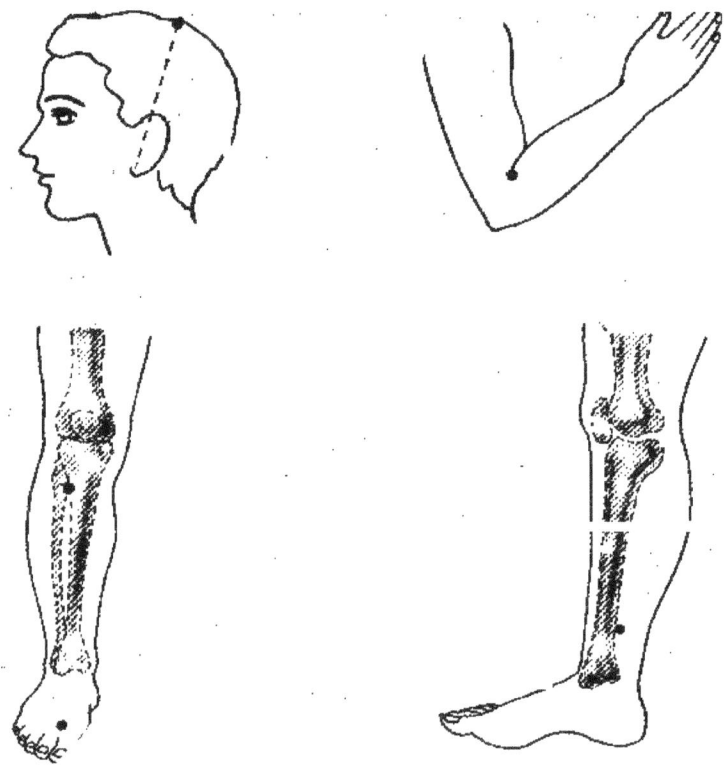

Note: All the points, except the first, are located on the right as well as the left side of the body.

Each point should be pressed rhythmically and firmly for about a minute, with the finger (or thumb) tip or the blunt end of a pencil. It is desirable to take this treatment in the lying posture. The treatment should be repeated 2 to 4 times a day.

Note: All the points, except the first, are located on the right as well as the left side of the body. Each point should be pressed rhythmically and firmly for about a minute, with the finger (or thumb) tip or the blunt end of a pencil. It is desirable to take this treatment in the lying posture. The treatment should be repeated 2 to 4 times a day.

ENDOCRINE GLANDS: Take treatment on all the endocrine glands-2 minutes on each point-3 times a day on both the palms/soles. These points will not only cure High Blood Pressure but will also improve the health in general. These points are nos.4 ,3 ,8, 38, 28, 25,29 and 11 to 15 as shown below. (all these points are related to Chakras)

Drink at least two glasses of gold/silver/copper charged water reduced from four glasses of water. If the use of gold and silver is not possible, drink at least copper + iron charged water two glasses reduced from four glasses of water.

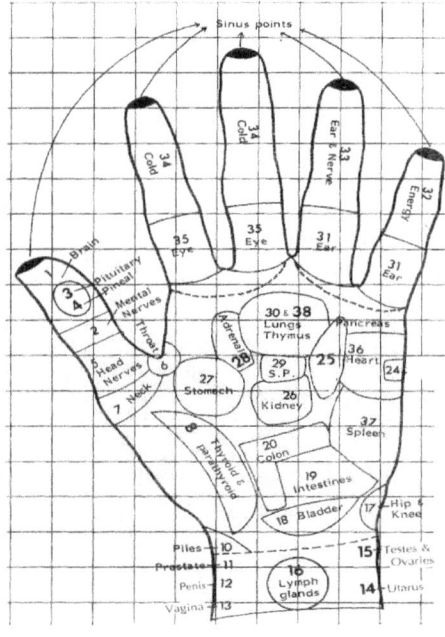

Right-Hand points of palms

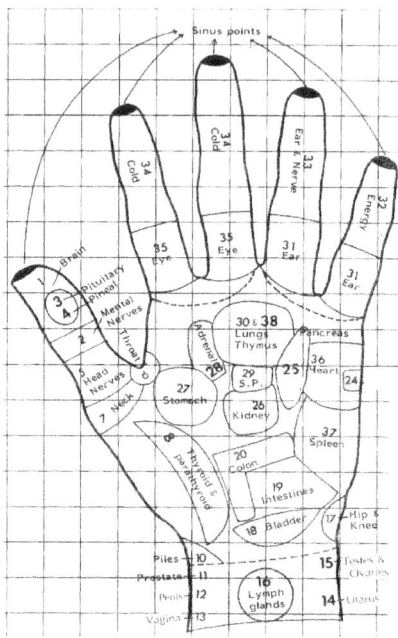

Left-Hand points of palms

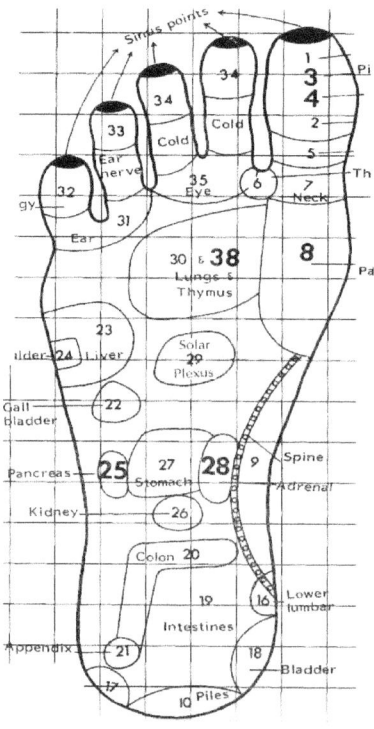

Right-Sole points of the soles

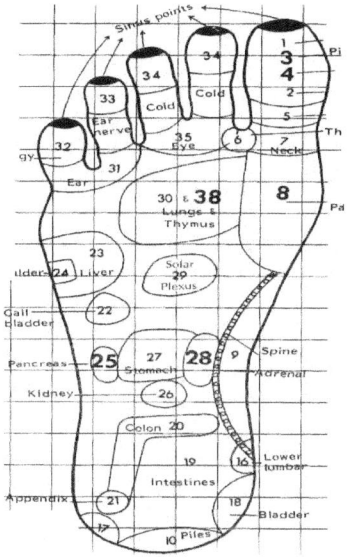

Left-leg Sole points connected with different organs and endocrine glands

As high B. P. leads to many other problems, it is utmost necessary to control it at the earliest. At the time of attack of high B. P. place the small finger in each ear and press them intermittently or shake them hard for 2 to 3 minutes. That will immediately lower the B. P. Also give treatment on Points Nos. 3-4-8-11 to 15-25 and 28. For long-term cure of this dreaded disease take the following treatment as mentioned earier:

- Stop/reduce salt and spices from the diet. Instead rock salt or black salt can be taken.
- Drink two cups of green juice adding thereto one tablespoonful of honey +1 teaspoon of Health Powder per cup.
- Drink at least one glass of fruit juice.
- Take action to reduce stress.

Shiatsu

Shiatsu treatment aim is to reestablish harmony. The body is capable of making appropriate adjustments and correcting our imbalanced conditions. Therefore for both hypertension and hypotension, shiatsu treatment is approximately the same. If the heart is beating too fast or too slow our treatment is about the same. Our body's adjustment mechanism, following natural patterns is the source of healing.

The most effective method for any aspect of heart disease is to give a complete shiatsu treatment. In general however, attention to the heart (HT) and heart governor (HG) channels on the arms is effective.

The area on the back between the shoulder blades near the spine (T3-T7) can be pressed. An abdominal massage and shiatsu on the lower back in the kidney region is helpful (T12-L4).Points UB 15 and UB 23 as shown in the picture below should be pressed.

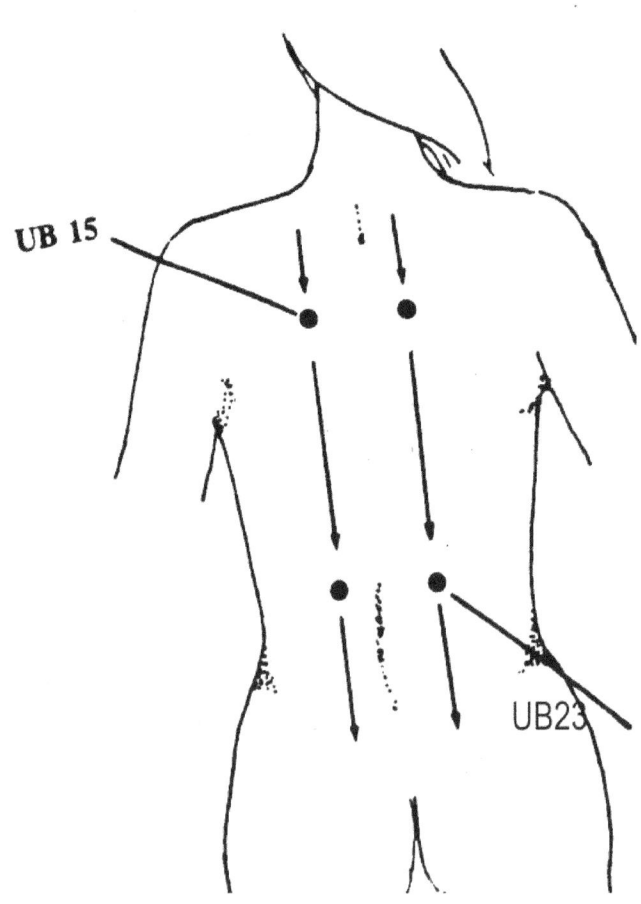

Annexure 1

Characteristics of A Type behaviour

A person with type A behaviour-

1. talks aggressively and hurriedly; he unnecessarily stresses or accentuates certain words while speaking and hurries the ends of the sentences,
2. always moves, walks and eats rapidly,

3. becomes impatient if events taking place in front of his eyes are slow; he strives to rapidly complete the sentence of others, thinking they speak too slowly or not to the point,

4. gets irritated and enraged if the vehicle in front is moving slowly,

5. gets impatient or irritated if he has to stand in a queue,

6. gets irritated if a work is being done slowly, while he thinks he could have done faster,

7. tries to accomplish more than one work at one time; he reads the newspaper while having his lunch or eats his morning breakfast while shaving,

8. prefers to go through the summary of a book instead of reading it fully,

9. always dwells in his own thoughts; while with others, he tries to bring the theme of the conversation to those that especially interest and intrigue him and if unable to accomplish this maneuver, pretends to listen but remains preoccupied with his own thoughts.

10. feels vaguely guilty if he has nothing to do even for a while; he just cannot enjoy a weekend or a vacation,

11. Attempts to schedule more and more in less and less time, leaving little room for unseen contingencies; in short, he suffers from a chronic sense of time-urgency,

12. feels challenged or jealous when in company of another 'type A' person,
13. unconsciously clinches his fists or jaws and grinds his teeth, while occupied in some work,

14. thinks that his success depends solely upon the pace of his work,

15. tries to accomplish most tasks in in hurry, avoids to employ a new idea or a new system and imagination and Creativity,

16. cannot remember the colour of furniture, most recently visited place; knows little about his neighbours, nearby shops or other places,

17. considers it to be a waste of time if he has to play with his children on returning home from work,

18. remains so engrossed in his activity that is unaware of things occurring around him,

19. has an extreme fascination for numbers; if a businessman, he is more interested in the figure of his income than in how he will use that money.

From above, it is clear that a 'type A' person considers life a battle, races against the clock and invites mental tension.

In an experiment, psychologists analysed the minds of thousands of college students to classify them into 'type A' and 'non type A' personalities. Thereafter, the psychologists predicted that most of the 'type A' students will develop high blood pressure over the years. This prediction turned out to be absolutely true. That 'non type A' students did not develop high blood pressure is only suggestive.

Annexure 2

Meditation Method

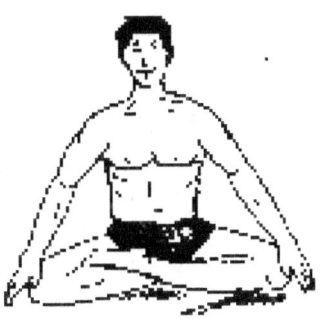

Schedule a few minutes each day to practice deep breathing. Also do it whenever you have some free time or when you are feeling stressed.

Sit with your back straight either in a chair or on the floor with your legs crossed in any posture that is comfortable. Relax your thinking and let the thoughts just drift off. Let your shoulders, then your arms, neck, and head become relaxed. Keep your eyes only half open with your gaze about five feet in front of you on the floor. Breathe only through your nose. Make your inhalation and exhalation the same length. Mentally, you can feel your whole body breathing, not just the nose and lungs. Practice this for as long as you like, up to twenty minutes at a time.

We cannot live without air for more than four minutes. With deep breathing, we get over seven times the normal volume of oxygen. This means that we enrich the blood with oxygen and vitality which, in turn, brings even more energy and essential life force.

The richness of the blood is the basis of the entire body's health, and the blood can be called rich only if it contains the necessary amount of oxygen and other nutrients. This comes from proper breathing, whole natural foods, and exercise.

Way of breathing is thus very important to maintain good health and avoid High Blood Pressure. Breathing should not be shallow but deep. We should practice proper breathing when we are tense as breathing helps to remove/ameliorate stress.

Bellows Breathing

This technique is a series of rapid, forceful abdominal exhalations followed by relaxed, natural inhalations. When you are feeling a little tired or sluggish, less than a minute
of bellows breathing may be especially helpful to increase your level of energy.

Here's how to do it:
Using the abdominal breathing technique, exhale fully and inhale fully, then exhale forcefully a small quantity of air. Move only your abdominal muscles. Increase the frequency of exhalations and inhalations to about two per second. After the fifteenth exhalation or if you experience any discomfort, resume breathing normally. You may wish to repeat this once or twice. End each session with a gentle, full exhalation, inhalation and exhalation.

Alternative Nostril Breathing

Your nose is lined with erectile tissue that expands and contracts during the day causing your nasal mucosa to swell and shrink. Although you probably are not aware of it, the flow of air through your nose shifts from one nostril to the other during the day as the lining of each nostril expands and contracts in a biological rhythm. For most people, the breath will flow predominantly through one nostril for about two hours, and then the predominance will begin to shift to the other nostril. Yoga texts state that this rhythm and alternating pattern is important in maintaining physiological and psychological equilibrium. Research has not yet been done to confirm or refute these concepts. We do know, for example, that the two hemispheres of the brain function somewhat differently. Maybe this, in turn, is reflected in your breathing.
The technique of alternate nostril breathing was developed to rebalance the equilibrium of breathing. Alternative nostril Breathing is an exceptionally powerful technique for calming and relaxing your mind and body.

Here is how to do it:

• Sit in a comfortable position and close your eyes.
• Exhale fully.
• Close off the right nostril with your thumb and inhale slowly through your left nostril. (Traditional yoga texts   instruct a person to make a gentle fist with the right hand, and then open only the thumb and the last two fingers. The side of the thumb is used to close off the right nostril and the

side of the ring finger is used to close off the left nostril. In practice though, do whatever is most comfortable for you.)

- Close off the left nostril and exhale through the right   nostril.
- Inhale through the right nostril.
- Close off the right nostril and exhale through the left

Continue this for about 10 minutes.

Annexure 3

Copper/Silver/Gold and Iron charged water:

It has been found that the following minerals are useful for treating diseases connected with the organs as shown below:

1. Copper: Useful for all diseases and problems connected with the nervous system e.g. high B.P., arthritis, polio, tension and leprosy.
2. Silver: Useful for diseases of the organs connected with digestive system and the urinary system.
3. Gold: Useful for disorders of the breathing system, lungs heart, brain and is a general tonic.
4. Iron: Proper quantity of iron in blood is utmost necessary because they carry oxygen and supplies it all over the body and thus increases stamina.

The charged water can be prepared as shown below

Take a pot of Pyrex glass, if possible; otherwise take a copper vessel, if readily available. In that case copper is not to be included while boiling. Otherwise stainless steel vessel even earthen pot can be used. Do not use Aluminum or brass vessel.

(1) Copper charged water: Put 60 grams of pure copper plate / ingots / wire or 6 to 8 copper coins in 4 glasses of water and boil it.

(2) Silver charged water: Put 30 to 60 grams of silver-pure bullion or pure coins.99.9 purity) in 4 glasses of water and boil it. Do not use silver ornaments.

(3) Gold charged water: 15 to 30 grams of gold pure bullion gold coin or ornaments (chain or bangles not enameled of 22 carat gold in 4 glasses of water and boil it).

(4) Iron charged water: (In case of deficiency of iron in blood anemia or during pregnancy) Put 60 grams of nonrusted piece of iron (nails, etc.) in 4 glasses of water and boil it.

All these metals can be put together in water, in the Proportion of gold 15 to 20 grams/silver 30 grams/copper (10 grams /iron 60 grams. It should be borne in mind that all metals put in the water are thoroughly cleaned and do not contain any dust or rust.

Boil away 25% of water i.e. retain 3 out of 4 glasses of water after boiling. Filter this water, keep it in a thermos if Possible and drink it lukewarm/ hot during the day. Drinking 1 glass of such water the first thing in the morning is very beneficial. When this water is reduced by 50%, it becomes medicine-best antibiotic and is a must in treatment of all serious diseases. In acute cases, this water may be boiled down to 1 glass or even half a glass. When you drink such concentrated water (i.e. when more than 60% water is boiled away e.g. 3 glasses of charged water reduced from 8 glasses).Avoid sour things like lemon, sour buttermilk, etc.

The charged water is found useful for good health. But it is a must for the treatment of any problems connected with the improper flow of the current of Bioelectricity i.e high B.P, polio, rheumatism, arthritis, paralysis and chronic diseases including cancer. Charged gold water has given wonderful results in cases of mental retardation, T.B and heart attack and is a good brain tonic.

Copper water is very useful for high Blood Pressure.

Other books by the author

Other books by the author

1. **How to heal and prevent diseases.**

This book informs how different foods can prevent and cure diseases.

2. Self-Examination

This book helps in diagnosis of diseases by inspection of body parts like nails, tongue, retina, ears and use of reflexology and Reiki. By these methods diseases can be diagnosed and prevented in initial stages.

www.ingramcontent.com/pod-product-compliance
Lightning Source LLC
Chambersburg PA
CBHW080644180526
45168CB00008B/3305